HOW TO KEEP A YOUTHFUL BODY

Susan Su

Copyright © 2023 *Susan Su*

CONTENTS

DISCLAIMER

SUSAN SU © 2023

DISCLAIMER

The author and publisher make no representation or warranties with respect to the accuracy, applicability, fitness, or completeness of the contents of this book; and assumes no responsibility for errors, omissions of the subject matter herein. All links are for information purposes only and are not warranted for content, accuracy, or any other implied or explicit purpose.

For practical advice books, like anything else in life, there are no guarantees of results made. Readers are cautioned to reply on their own judgment about their individual circumstances to act accordingly.

1. INTRODUCTION

We're born, we grow old, we die. It's a rhythm long considered inevitable. The average life span for men and women increase dramatically. The life expectancy for men today is 84.3 years; for women, it is 86.6 years. One in four 65-year-olds today will live past the age of 90, and one in ten will live past 95. As of this writing, the oldest person alive is 119, a woman named Kane Tanaka who has lived through over a century of history's momentous events, including the Spanish Flu – the last global pandemic before Covid-19. Better health care, improved hygiene, greater emphasis on a healthy lifestyle, adequate nutritious food, better medical care, and reduced child mortality all contribute to the longevity. As men and women are living to older age nowadays, everyone wants to keep a youthful body as aging. So know how to keep a youthful body is important

Aging is something we all do, such as memory loss, wrinkles, and lean muscle loss, but understand very little about. Not a lot of people really understands what aging is, why it happens, and whether we can actually slow or stop it.

The book uncovers the reason cause aging, and then how to keep a youthful body to slow aging process. It covers topics from what is aging, different type of aging, different theories on the reason of aging, the aging process and how to slow aging and have a youthful body.

When the Human Genome Project was completed in 2003, the field of ageing expected remarkable findings from "cracking" the genetic code, the "genetic" era of health. In the last 15 years, a new era appeared, called the "epigenetic" era. This is the science of how our environment influences the activity of our genes. Lifestyle can switch certain genes on and others off. Choices made about nutrition are the most powerful environmental factors that influence gene activity, followed by fitness, quality of sleep, toxins including smoking, and stress. Our genes may load the "longevity and health" gun, but lifestyle pulls the trigger, or not.

2. WHAT CAUSE AGING

Aging refers to the physiological changes we experience during our lifespan that comes with age, such as memory loss, wrinkles, and lean muscle loss. It is the progressive accumulation of changes with time that are associated with or responsible for the ever-increasing susceptibility to disease and death. Aging is an unavoidable process of deterioration that can be modulated but not completely stopped by evolution. It's an inevitable part of life.

The sum of the deleterious free radical reactions going on continuously throughout the cells and tissues constitutes the aging process or is a major contributor to it. The common denominator that underlies all modern theories of biological aging is change in molecular structure and, hence, function. In other words, it is the progressive damage to these structures and functions that we perceive and characterize as aging.

Aging is a result of a significant number of causes. There are currently more than 300 theories on why we age, and experts are learning more every day. No single process can explain all the changes of aging. Some theories claim that aging is caused by injuries from ultraviolet light over time, wear and tear on the body, or byproducts of metabolism. Other theories view aging as a predetermined process controlled by genes. Many also believe that free radicals and oxidative stress play an insignificant role in aging. Aging is the generated by multiple causes damage to the structures and functions of the molecules, cells, organs, etc., of an organism. Such causes of aging include but are not limited to oxidative stress, glycation, telomere shortening, side reactions, enzyme infidelity, mutations, aggregation of proteins, free radicals, ROS, and oxidative stress etc.

The factors caused aging can be categorized into two types, intrinsic and extrinsic. Intrinsic aging is a genetically predetermined process that occurs naturally. Extrinsic aging is a result of outside factors, such as where you live, your stress levels, and your lifestyle habits (like smoking). Cellular aging is due to intrinsic factors. It's related to the biological aging of cells. Cells are the basic building blocks of the body. Your cells are programmed to divide, multiply, and perform basic biological functions. But the more cells divide, the older they get. In turn, cells eventually lose their ability to function properly. Cellular damage accumulated over time also increases as cells get older. This makes the cell less healthy, causing biological processes to fail. Damage-related and environmental aging is related to extrinsic factors. It refers to how our surroundings and lifestyle affect how we age. This includes factors like: air pollution, tobacco smoke, alcohol consumption, malnutrition, ultraviolet radiation (UV) exposure. Over time, these factors can damage our cells and contribute to aging.

Agents of different types also synergize in causing damage. Damage resulting from the action of a certain cause depends also on the action of other causes. Significant damage (aging) occurs when the force (level) of more than one cause of aging increases substantially. The rate of generation of damage, the rate of aging, increases dramatically with time when the causes of aging (structural and functional damage) interact synergistically. Early in life, the assurance systems function optimally and therefore the rate of aging is slow and almost flat. The rate of aging increases when the rate of damage generation increases and the assurance mechanisms start failing later in life. In principle, a substantial increase in health and lifespan might be achieved if we manage to substantially restore the function of one or more failed assurance mechanisms.

3. VARIOUS AGING THEORIES

While aging is caused by multiple processes that interact and overlap with each other, rather than one reason. There are many aging theories, some of the most prominent theories are as following.

1. **Programmed theories of aging**

It says that people are designed to age and that our cells have a predetermined lifespan that's encoded into our bodies. Also called active, or adaptive, aging theories, they include:

- **Gene theory.** This theory suggests that specific genes turn "on" and "off" over time, causing aging.

- **Endocrine theory.** Aging is caused by changes in hormones, which are produced by the endocrine system.

- **Immunological theory.** Also called the autoimmune theory, it says the immune response is designed to decline. The result is disease and aging.

2. **Genetic theory of aging**

The genetic theory proposes that aging primarily depends on genetics. In other words, our life expectancy is regulated by the genes we got from our parents. Genetic theories include:

- **Telomere theory.** Telomeres protect the ends of chromosomes as they multiply. Over time, telomeres shorten, which is associated with disease and aging.

- **Programmed senescence theory.** Cellular senescence occurs when cells stop dividing and growing, but don't die.

- **Stem cell theory.** Stem cells can turn into other cells, which helps repair tissue and organs. But the function of stem cells declines over time, potentially contributing to aging.

- **Longevity gene theory.** This is the idea that certain genes extend lifespan.

3. **Evolutionary theory of aging:**

According to evolutionary theories, aging is based on natural selection which refers to the adaptive traits of an organism. These traits can help the organism adjust to their environment, so they're more likely to survive. Organisms begin aging after they have reached their peak of reproduction and have passed down adaptive traits. Evolutionary theories include:

- **Mutation accumulation.** This theory presumes that random mutations accumulate later in life.

- **Antagonistic pleiotropy**. According to this theory, genes that promote fertility early in life have negative effects later on.

- **Disposable soma theory.** When more metabolic resources are directed toward reproduction, the less is put toward DNA repair. The result is cell damage and aging.

4. **Biochemical theory of aging**

   These reactions occur naturally and continuously throughout life. This theory is rooted in various concepts, including:

   - **Advanced glycation end products (AGEs).** AGEs develop when fats or protein are exposed to sugar. High levels may lead to oxidative stress, which speeds up aging.

   - **Heat shock response**. Heat shock proteins protect cells from stress, but their response decreases as we age.

   - **Damage accumulation.** Normal chemical reactions damage DNA, proteins, and metabolites over time.

5. **Error theories of aging**

   Error theories, or damage theories, are the opposite of programmed theories. They hypothesize that aging is caused by cellular changes that are random and unplanned. Error theories of aging include:

- **Wear and tear theory.** This is the idea that cells break down and become damaged over time. But critics argue that it doesn't account for the body's ability to repair.

- **Genome instability theory**. Aging happens because the body loses its ability to repair DNA damage.

- **Cross-linkage theory**. Aging is due to the buildup of cross-linked proteins, which damages cells and slows biological functions.

- **Rate-of-living theory.** Proponents of this theory say that an organism's rate of metabolism determines its lifespan.

- **Free radical theory**. This theory suggests that aging is due to the buildup of oxidative stress, which is caused by free radicals.

- **Mitochondrial theory**. As a variation of the free radical theory, this theory says that mitochondrial damage releases free radicals and causes aging.

4. AGING PROCESS

Growing old is unavoidable. No matter what you do, your body will change in a number of key ways. For example, by the time a person turns 20, lung tissues will begin to lose their elasticity, the muscles around the rib cage will start to deteriorate, and the overall lung function will gradually begin to diminish. Similarly, the production of digestive enzymes will begin to slow as we age, which affects how nutrients are absorbed into the body and the types of food we can digest without difficulty. As women approach menopause, vaginal fluids will decrease and sexual tissues will start to atrophy due to the loss of estrogen. In men, lean muscles will thin and sperm production will diminish due to decreases in testosterone levels. Blood vessels also lose their flexibility as we age. In people who are sedentary and eat poor diets, the loss of elasticity paired with the accumulation of fatty deposits can lead to atherosclerosis ("hardening of the arteries"). There are main four types of aging:

Cellular Aging: A cell can replicate about 50 times before the genetic material is no longer able to be copied accurately. This replication failure is referred to as cellular senescence during which the cell loses its functional characteristics. The accumulation of senescent cells is the hallmark of cellular aging, which in turn translates to biological aging. The more damage done to cells by free radicals and environmental factors, the more cells need to replicate and the more rapidly that cellular senescence develops. The cells in our bodies take quite a beating throughout our lifetimes. Environmental factors, such as ultraviolet rays, poor diet, and alcohol, as well as psychological factors including stress, are putting our cells at risk of significant damage.

Hormonal Aging: Hormones play a huge role in aging. Over time, the output of many hormones will begin to diminish, leading to changes in the skin (such as wrinkles and the loss of elasticity) and a loss of muscle tone, bone density, and sex drive.

Accumulative Damage: Aging caused by accumulative damage (i.e., "wear and tear") is about the external factors that can build up over time. Exposure to toxins, UV radiation, unhealthy foods, and pollution can just some of the things that can take a toll on the body. Over time, these external factors can directly damage DNA in cells (in part by exposing them to excessive or persistent inflammation). The accumulated damage can undermine the body's ability to repair itself, promoting rapid aging.

Metabolic Aging: As you go about your day, your cells are constantly turning food into energy, which produces byproducts—some of which can be harmful to the body. The process of metabolization, while essential, can cause progressive damage to cells, a phenomenon referred to as metabolic aging. Some experts believe that slowing down the metabolic process through practices such as calorie restriction may slow aging in humans

5. HOW TO SLOW AGING

Aging cannot be avoided. With that said, there are several things you can do to mitigate the environmental factors that influence aging:

☐ **Eat well.** Avoid Added sugar, salt, and saturated fat , increase your intake of fruits, vegetables, whole grains, low-fat dairy, and lean meat and fish. Eat a heathy diet.

☐ **Read labels**. Check the label of the packaged foods to ensure that you limit sodium intake to under 1,500 milligrams (mg) per day, the sugar intake to around 25 mg per day, and saturated fat intake to less than 10% of daily calories.

☐ **Stop smoking.** Quitting cigarettes improves circulation and blood pressure while drastically reducing risk of cancer.

☐**Exercise.** Exercise Keep your muscles and bones strong. The recommended exercise requirements for good health is roughly 30 minutes of moderate to strenuous exercise 5 days per week. Even so, 15 minutes of moderate activity per day can improve longevity compared to no exercise. Dancing may help to relieve the appearance of inflammatory skin conditions. Regular yoga practice can help reduce the appearance of premature ageing. Even meditation can help flush away toxins in your skin as you breathe in the good and breathe out the bad.

☐**Socialize.** Socialization keeps us psychologically engaged and may help influence longevity. Maintain good, healthy relationships with others. Stay connected to the ones you love, and make it a point to meet new people.

☐ **Get ample sleep.** Chronic sleep deprivation is linked to poorer health and shorter life spans. By improving your sleep hygiene and getting around 7 to 8 hours of sleep per night, you may not only feel better but live longer.

☐ **Reduce stress.** Chronic stress and anxiety can be damaging to your body as they trigger the release of an inflammatory stress hormone called cortisol. Learning to control stress with relaxation techniques and mind-body therapies may help alleviate the indirect inflammatory pressure placed on cells.

☐**Maintain healthy DNA.** Vitamin A helps to control how cells divide, grow and mature. So, if the cells are healthy, you will have healthy DNA too. By supplementing your diet with vitamin A, whether it's in the food you eat or the vitamins you take, you can help maintain healthy DNA.

6. HEALTHY HABITS TO STAY YOUNG

Experts agree that "staying young" begins in the mind. Stressing about life's many highs and lows can cause more than a few grey hairs; surges of hormones adrenaline and cortisol can cause high blood pressure and stress the heart. If you want to increase your longevity and keep yourself young at heart for years to come, try these expert-approved strategies on how to stay looking and feeling young. The following tips are key elements in how to stay young and make the most of your life every day.

1.Take a Mindful Break: Studies show that stress causes physical changes in the body that can accelerate aging. Surges of the hormones adrenaline and cortisol cause blood pressure to rise and the heart to beat faster. These days, when stressors seem unrelenting (a steady stream of job pressures, traffic jams, money problems), chronic doses of adrenaline and cortisol can take a heavy toll on your physical and emotional health. One of the most effective way to reduce stress is to meditate. Try your best to sit in a quiet place with your eyes closed, relaxing your jaw and shoulders, connecting to your breath, emptying your mind, and staying in the present moment for ten to 20 minutes each day. Do yoga, or something active and repetitive (such as mindful running) instead. Focus on your breathing and how your feet land with each stride — and get your to-do list out of your head.

2. Eat More Fat: Omega-3 fatty acids (found in salmon, walnuts, and seeds) help stabilize your mood, maintain bone strength, and help prevent visible signs of aging by reducing inflammation in the body. It also boosts the ability of the body's enzymes to pull fat out of storage --from your hips, say--and use it as energy. It also keeps you healthy and your skin radiant. You need two grams of omega-3 fatty acids a day. Eat plenty of fatty fish such as wild salmon (a 3-ounce serving has 6.9 grams), as well as walnuts (one-half ounce has 9.2 grams). If you aren't getting enough omega-3s from your diet, consider taking fish oil supplements.

3.Get Moving: Not only can regular exercise help you tone muscles, build healthier bones, and boost your mood, but it can also help you think clearly. Walking for just 10 minutes a day lowers your risk of Alzheimer's by 40 percent. Physical conditioning reduces stress and anxiety, which wipe out your memory bank. Make time for three 20-minute workouts a week. You can also run, bike, swim, dance — simply do whatever you enjoy most. Doing whatever physical activity you love most is one great way to stay young.

4.Find Love: And we don't only mean romantically! Love can be found in all forms – in friends, in family, in pets, and hobbies. Passion is a powerful drug, the ability to embrace life in all its variety. Rekindle romance with your partner, join a club or group with common interests, take a painting class, or invite others to walk with you. You'll find yourself feeling more energized and your self-esteem will get a boost. Anyone who's ever fallen head over heels or discovered an activity that makes them eager to jump out of bed in the morning knows that passion is a powerful drug and the central motivation of all human activity. The ability to embrace life boosts self-esteem, fuels the immune system, and improves cardiovascular health. Passion in bed can be particularly beneficial: Getting it on triggers the release of oxytocin (AKA the "love hormone"), and has been shown to reduce feelings of stress and anxiety. Banish boredom and isolation at all costs. Rekindle the flames with your partner. Or discover a new love in the form of a mental or physical pursuit: Take up painting, join a book club, start a running program. Do what make you feel energized and happy.

5. Try/do Yoga: As a mind-body exercise, yoga pairs conscious breathing with physical movement. This gentle exercise can increase energy, and improve posture, flexibility, and mood. Deep oxygenating breath can help eliminate toxins in the body, prevent illness, and make skin glow. Regardless of a person's age or experience level, yoga is another great way to stay young. Through conscious yoga breathing, you become aware of the connection between mind and body. Yogic breathing can help decrease stress and anxiety. Yoga poses are designed to work the inside of your body as well as the outside, which helps rejuvenate the digestive system, the reproductive system, and even the immune system. Yoga is like wringing your body out like a washcloth. It's one of the best ways to keep things moving. Practice yoga or other mind-body activities at least twice a week to give yourself an energy boost, help build bone mass, and de-stress.

6.Eat More Fruit: Superfruits like pomegranates, goji berries, and blueberries have rich sources of Vitamins C and E, and antioxidants, which help lower cholesterol and blood pressure, reduce joint inflammation, and may help reduce the risk of Alzheimer's disease. Goji berry has an abundant source of carotenoids, a beneficial type of antioxidant. This little nutritional powerhouse also contains more iron than spinach; 18 amino acids; calcium; magnesium; zinc;

selenium; and vitamins B1, B2, B6, and E. The goji berry stimulates the release of human growth hormone, a natural substance in the body that improves your ability to sleep, helps you look younger, reduces fat, improves memory, boosts libido, and enhances the immune system.To benefit from these antioxidants, try snacking on dried goji berries, or ask your doctor about concentrated goji berry supplements, or try a pomegranate-infused skin serum to achieve a skin-plumping glow. Pomegranate juice has been found to lower cholesterol and blood pressure, possibly delay the onset of atherosclerosis, and potentially help reduce the risk of Alzheimer's disease; researchers believe it may also help prevent some forms of cancer from starting or progressing. Pomegranates can also protect the skin from damage caused by UV rays.

7.Play Brain Games, Do Mental Aerobics

Brain games like crossword puzzles and sudoku can help prevent cognitive decline, strengthen the mind, and improve memory. You can find many brain games on Lumosity. Or you can find any number of brain game workbooks involving numbers, sequences, and wordplay at your nearby bookstore or online.

8. Spend Time Outdoors: Fresh air and sunshine revitalize the mind and body. Sunlight triggers the release of serotonin, a chemical in the brain that improves sleep, appetite, and digestion. Whether working in the garden, reading in the park, or chatting with a neighbor "over the fence," spending time outdoors in the fresh air can be a great way to stay young.

9.Treat Yourself: It's important to take care of yourself, no matter your age. Get a massage. Buy a new outfit. Bring home a bouquet of flowers. Do whatever brings a smile to your face, raises your spirits, and reignites that inner spark of youth.

10.Drink Red Wine (in Moderation): A substance found in the skin of grapes, had longer average lifespans than those not given the resveratrol. Resveratrol reduced the risk of diabetes and liver problems in mice, leading to a significant decline in obesity-related deaths. Red wine can diminish brain damage caused by stroke by as much as 40 percent. And grape-seed procyanidins, found in red wine, help reduce arterial clogging, resulting in lower blood cholesterol levels and a reduction in deaths from heart disease.

11.Sip Green Tea: Green tea is an amazing compound in terms of blocking the signaling network that is linked with the progression of cancer. Drinking at least one cup a day can help keep your brain sharp as you get older.

12.Prioritize Sleep: Consistently getting poor sleep not only makes you feel exhausted but also has a serious impact on your health. Insufficient sleep ups the risk of developing diabetes and cardiovascular disease — and more importantly, it can impact your life expectancy. Yes, even getting *too much* sleep can impact your health: Research shows snoozing for 8 to 9 hours or more is linked with a greater risk of coronary heart disease, stroke, cardiovascular disease, and type 2 diabetes.

13. Try the Mediterranean Diet: In addition to supporting heart health, reducing the risk of cancer, and preventing cognitive decline, the Mediterranean diet may help protect your telomeres, DNA sequences that sit at the ends of chromosomes and protect them from damage. Telomere length is considered a biomarker of aging: Shorter telomeres are linked with a lower life expectancy and increased risk of developing chronic disease. While telomere length typically decreases with age, this shortening can be sped up by oxidative stress and inflammation, according to the researchers.

Sticking to a Mediterranean diet may help fend off that damage. The primary foods involved in the Mediterranean diet — i.e. fruits, vegetables, and nuts — are known to have antioxidant and anti-inflammatory effects, meaning they may protect against the oxidative stress and inflammation that can cause telomere shortening. Load your plate with fruits, veggies, nuts, legumes, unrefined grains, and fish; cook with olive oil in place of butter and vegetable oil; and keep your consumption of dairy and meat to a minimum.

14.Have more sex: having sex frequently could help you live longer.

7. TIPS FOR AGING GRACEFULLY

1. Do something you enjoy every day. When you immerse yourself in things you enjoy, you can't wait to do them again. Then you do them again, and again and again, and the enjoyment continues

2. Work at friendships. Friendships are fuel, providing energy, love and feeding your emotions.

3. Congratulate yourself. Everyone has accomplishments: celebrate them and use them as inspiration for new ones.

4. Embrace change. Life is change. Living for it can create adventures you never thought possible.

5. Learn. Exercise your brain continually.

6. Know yourself. You know best what you like and don't like, and you have the power to emphasize the good.

7. Make your home your special place by personalizing it and making it comfortable.

8. Realize that opportunities often express themselves in ways we'd never imagine.

9. Get a massage frequently. Touch feels good and it's so relaxing.

10. Be gentle with yourself. Listen to your own inner voices and senses and do what makes you feel best.

11. Share happiness. Make a point to spread joy whenever possible. It feels good to make someone else feel good.

12. Eat with friends and family. Prepare food together. Eat the things you like.

13. Eat smartly, but every once in awhile line up a row of warm chocolate chip cookies and dip them in milk.

14. Get sufficient rest. Living takes work; we all need a break. Take one whenever you need to.

15. Laugh and cry. But laugh a lot more. It feels good by releasing endorphins – the body's natural feel-good chemicals.

16. Each morning before you get out of bed thank the Lord for 5 things for which you are grateful. It's a nice way to start the day, and you'll find yourself thinking about a lot more than 5.

17. Take control of how you react to things. Little things can really bring you down if you let them. But you don't have to let them.

18. Smile a lot.

19. Pray daily.

20. Spend time with other generations. You can learn something new from someone of any age.

21. Write. Write a letter, a blog, a poem or a journal. Writing helps you think, express who you are, and generate new ideas.

22. Embrace technology. The internet can take you places you'd never otherwise see or experience.

23. Dress in current styles. By adding a trendy piece to a classic outfit, you will look and feel good.

24. Travel. A trip to the mall, theater, a sports event or even a different state or country, little and big adventures can produce wonderful results.

25. Exercise. It feels good to get those endorphins jumping.

26. Drink and eat in moderation.

27. Get a yearly medical checkup. While it's no guarantee you'll live longer, it can help you catch health issues early and fend off other potential health problems.

28. Get a pet. Animals can be great companions.

29. Simplify. Start with cleaning a closet. Next simplify other parts of your life.

30. Surround yourself with people who lift you up rather than bring you down.

31. Don't try to be everything to everyone. It's impossible.

32. Always have something to solve. Making progress feels good and often it helps someone else and brings happiness.

33. Embrace the joys of old age. You're smarter; you're more experienced and you have more time to do the things you enjoy.

34. Practice acceptance. Know that there's a very good chance that your mobility will lessen as you age. Think about how you will deal with that so that when that time comes, you can still live fully.

35. Create milestones and work toward them. No matter how big or small, the journey is a growing experience.

36. Realize that although your body deteriorates, your spirit grows stronger if you allow it.

37. Do not let yourself be diminished by anyone. You are you. No one else is, and that's darn important.

38. When you need supportive services, partner with a senior services provider that empowers you to enjoy life on your terms. Pre-

plan so that you have peace of mind that you will have the help you need in an environment you desire.

39. Value your body. If you do, you'll participate in less risky behavior that could harm your health.

40. Treat others with respect and dignity. You'll find respect and dignity come back to you.

41. Have someone you can tell anything.

42. Maintain muscle mass, it will protect you from falling.

43. Cut down or eliminate multi-tasking. Research shows people don't do it very well, and it often just causes undue stress.

44. Walk. take 5,000 to 10,000 steps every day.

45. Keep your weight at a healthy level.

46. Don't fear aging.

47. Grow to the very last breath.

8. HOW TO STAY YOUNGER

Trying to live longer is a great goal, but those extra years won't mean much if you're not feeling healthy and energetic. So why not try to help your body act younger than your chronological age, by following a few basic steps towards a longevity lifestyle? Making these changes today, to make your body function in a more youthful and resilient way, months, or years from now.

1. **Quit smoking:** Numerous studies have chronicled the toll tobacco takes on the overall well-being and health status of both men and women. More specifically, continuing a heavy smoking habit past the age of 40 has been shown to chop as much as a decade off your life. It can worsen many age-related diseases like heart disease and diabetes. Smoking also causes premature skin aging, making you look older. Stopping smoking will do more for your longevity and health in general — than any other change you make.

2. **Maintain a Healthy weight:** Too much fat on the body predisposes one to many serious conditions like heart disease, stroke, diabetes, and cancer; and link to metabolic syndrome, which includes symptoms like high blood sugar and elevated blood pressure, or hypertension. Finding out the right number of calories

you should consume each day and tackling a moderate and sustainable weight loss plan will make it easier to remain active and mobile, and help your body's functional, or biological age, stay as low as possible in the months, and years, to come.

3. **Stay Active:** The benefits of being physically active are numerous: better cardiovascular health, lower risk of cancer and diabetes, improved stress management, and better longevity. Whether walking, swimming, running, or some other activity appeals to you, stay active to ward off disease, keep your bones strong, and your life long!

4. **Eat an Anti-Aging Diet:** Eating a well-balanced diet based on fruits, vegetables, lean protein, plenty of low-mercury fish, whole grains, and moderate amounts of healthy fats, has consistently been linked to better longevity. While supplementing your diet with vitamins and minerals might help compensate for some missing components, most nutritionists advise getting your nutrients from food. Making healthy food choices, in the proper amounts (to avoid obesity), is a hedge against disease and a smart way to keep your body acting young

5. **Manage Your Stress:** Stress has many physiological effects, including raising your level of cortisol, a stress hormone that can contribute to cardiovascular conditions, dangerous belly fat, depression and poorer resistance to disease. Stress relief contribute to longevity. Mindfulness meditation, self-hypnosis, or even just smiling more, to manage your daily stress level.

6. **Stay Social:** Another important aspect of a longevity lifestyle is being part of a larger social network, with the support of friends and family. Staying connected and remaining integrated within their community were some of the most significant predictors of greater longevity. If not all members of your social circle are up to the task, pick your team: a few friends and confidants can help you bear difficult times, and cope with hardship, more easily — factors that will help your immune system keep you healthy.

You don't need to drastically change your daily habits to make improvements in these areas. Focus on progress, not perfection, and over time, your body will be healthier and behaving like that of a younger person.

10. EXERCISE TO LOSE WEIGHT

Healthy and consistent nutrition is a huge part, but without exercise, you aren't able to achieve the actual body shape you want. Calorie restriction without effective exercise will just leave you in a saggy human shell, you simply go from being overweight to being a skinny fat person.

By lacking the muscle and bone structure not to mention a healthy mind-set to hold yourself with strength or confidence you don't feel empowered or positive about your body because underneath the smaller-sized clothing are still the side effects of being overweight. The flabby flesh and loose skin, wobbly bits and lack of muscle tone are still lurking underneath. The answer to these problem is… the gift of **EXERCISE**! Yes, heart pumping, body moving, endorphin-releasing, muscle strengthening and enjoyable exercise!

The way to shape the body is through effective weight resistance exercise. Starvation and deprivation will never get you the results you crave!

Exercise can take many forms, including cardiovascular exercise, strength training, flexibility training, and balance training. Some common examples of exercise include running, cycling, swimming, weightlifting, yoga, and Pilates.

Exercise is not directly responsible for generating new cells in the body, but it can stimulate the process of cell growth and regeneration by promoting the production of certain hormones and growth factors. It has numerous other health benefits that contribute to overall cellular health and function. Regular exercise has been shown to promote the growth and repair of various tissues, including muscles, bones, and organs. When you exercise, your body responds by increasing blood flow, oxygen, and nutrient delivery to the cells, which can promote cell growth and repair.

Additionally, exercise has been shown to stimulate the production of growth hormone and testosterone, both of which play a key role in cellular growth and regeneration. The actual process of cell division and proliferation is a complex biological process that is regulated by many factors, including genetics, nutrition, and environmental factors. Therefore, while exercise can promote cellular growth and regeneration, it is just one of many factors that contribute to the overall health and function of your cells.

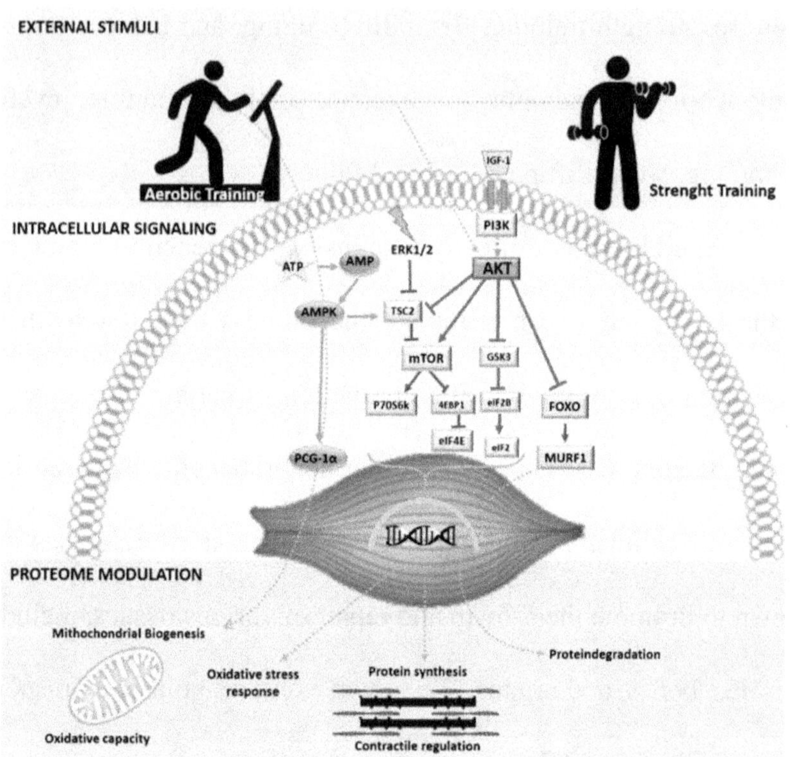

Another benefit of exercise is that it helps the brain make new neurons. In the hippocampus, a brain structure key to learning and memory, there are cells known as neural progenitors that can give rise to new brain cells. Neurogenes in adulthood helps keep certain cognitive skills sharp, including the ability to learn about the physical environment and remember how to navigate it. Regular exercise showed brain benefits in the memory tests also had markers of neurogenesis.

During exercise, the body experiences a variety of physical stresses, such as mechanical stress, oxidative stress, and metabolic stress. These stresses can activate various signaling pathways that stimulate the production of growth factors, such as insulin-like growth factor 1 (IGF-1), vascular endothelial growth factor (VEGF), and brain-derived neurotrophic factor (BDNF). These growth factors can promote the growth and proliferation of cells, including muscle cells, bone cells, and brain cells.

Exercise has also been shown to increase the production of stem cells, which are special cells that can differentiate into different types of cells. Stem cells play a critical role in tissue regeneration and repair, and regular exercise may help to maintain the pool of stem cells in the body. Furthermore, exercise can improve circulation and oxygen delivery to cells, which supports their function and promote their growth and regeneration. This is particularly important for cells with limited blood supply, such as cartilage and intervertebral discs.

In Summary, Regular exercise has numerous health benefits, including:

- Improving cardiovascular health by strengthening the heart and reducing the risk of heart disease, stroke.
- Boosting immune function by increasing the production of antibodies and white blood cells.
- Improving mental health by reducing symptoms of depression, anxiety, and stress.
- Improving bone density and reducing the risk of osteoporosis.
- Reducing the risk of certain types of cancer, such as colon and breast cancer.
- Reducing the risk of obesity and metabolic disorders, such as diabetes.
- Improving sleep quality and quantity.

11. *WALKING, THE QUINTESSENTIAL TO STAY ACTIVE!*

WHAT HAPPENS TO
YOUR BODY
on a Walk

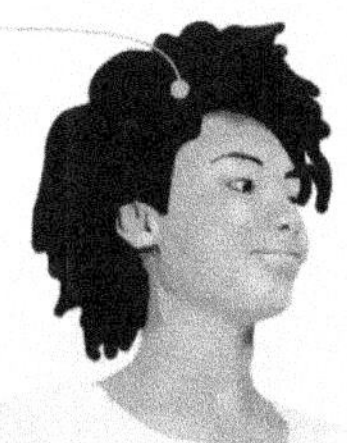

BRAIN

Walking boosts blood flow to the brain, decreases stress hormones and releases endorphins, improving mood, lowering depression and reducing the risk of cognitive decline.

MUSCLES

Walking up and down hills increases the activation of the hip, knee and ankle muscles; the steeper the grade, the bigger the benefit.

BONES

Like other weight-bearing activities, walking can help maintain bone health.

WEIGHT

Walking at least 30 minutes per day is linked to lower body weight, body fat and waist circumference.

BLOOD

Walking can help reduce insulin resistance, keeping blood sugar levels balanced and energy levels even.

HEART

Increasing your heart rate improves blood flow and helps your heart pump more efficiently, reducing the risk of cardiovascular disease.

DIGESTION

A post-meal walk can help food move through your digestive system, reducing bloating and digestion problems.

JOINTS

Movement increases the circulation of synovial fluid around the joints, providing essential lubrication and nutrients to the cartilage, the tissues that act as a cushion between bones.

SUSAN SU © 2023

Walking is more likely to be sustained due to the ease with which it can be incorporated into an individual's life. One of the major benefits of regular walking is how it can be adapted to activities of daily living such as commuting to and from work, or whilst taking phone calls. Start by walking more to increase your activity levels.

Research shows that 2-minute bouts of light to moderate walking every 20 minutes after a meal has significant reductions (around 24-30%) in blood glucose levels after eating. Furthermore, other important benefits of simply walking for 10-30 minutes 3 days weekly include improved sleep quality, stress relief, improved mood, cardiorespiratory fitness, improved energy and stamina and reduced fatigue.

12. HALLELUJAH DIET

Hallelujah Diet is a plant-based diet that emphasizes the consumption of raw and minimally processed plant-based foods, with an emphasis on consuming a large portion of these foods in their raw state. The diet was developed by Rev. George Malkmus, who found that the diet helped him overcome cancer in the 1970s. Hallelujah Diet has numerous health benefits, including weight loss, improved digestion, increased energy, and reduced risk of chronic diseases such as heart disease and cancer. Hallelujah Diet can be a great choice for promoting youthfulness, as it can provide many of the key nutrients that support healthy skin, hair, and overall vitality.

A vegan diet eliminates all animal products, which are the primary sources of saturated fat and cholesterol in the diet. This can help lower blood cholesterol levels and reduce the risk of heart disease. Many plant-based foods such as legumes, tofu, tempeh, seitan, and some grains and vegetables are good sources of protein. A vegan diet is typically high in fibre, which is important for digestive health and can also help lower the risk of chronic diseases such as colon cancer and heart disease. A vegan diet also has a lower carbon footprint than a diet that includes animal products, making it a more environmentally sustainable choice. While a vegan diet can be healthy, it's important to ensure that you are getting adequate amounts of key nutrients such as vitamin B12, iron, calcium, and omega-3 fatty acids.

Following a vegan diet may very well support the ageing process better compared to other diets that focus on less nutrient-dense foods. It is important to note, however, that this may be due to a higher intake of fruits, veggies, legumes, nuts, and seeds- as opposed to exclusively the vegan diet. The key to aging well seems to be more about achieving adequate nutrient intake, avoidance of nutritional deficiencies, and an emphasis on nutrient-dense foods. Certain kinds of animal products (like cured meats containing nitrites) have been linked to age-related diseases like Parkinson's and Alzheimer's, there's a chance that eating a vegan diet devoid of these products could help you stay sharp as you get older, too. A vegan diet may help you look younger and get around many of the aches, pains, and degenerative diseases that affect us as we get older instead. A vegan diet can contribute to a boost in metabolism given its high fibre content. These insoluble fibre compounds trigger the body to work harder to digest them, causing an increase in energy expenditure. This will increase metabolism, promoting a boost in the calorie-burning process. Over time, this process can prevent excess weight gain and improve metabolism. The vegan diet is high in antioxidants and anti-inflammatory compounds, which play a key role in helping prevent the development of chronic illnesses.

As we age, the prevalence of chronic illnesses increases, adding to the deteriorating factor of ageing. Antioxidants, found in most vegetable sources, help prevent cell damage caused by free radicals. This, in turn, prevents further inflammation and further cell damage associated with ageing. A diet rich in antioxidants, like the vegetarian and vegan diet, can help prevent and stabilize cellular damage that occurs in the process of ageing.

Chronic disease prevention is a key component of aging better. Adequate fibre is associated with improved digestive health and reduced risk of heart disease and Type 2 Diabetes. Vegan diets increase your lifespan by giving you more fibre, plant protein and antioxidants to eat. Eating vegan also reduces red meat intake which can decrease the risk of cardiovascular disease. A vegan diet can also reduce your risks of osteoarthritis. Of course, you'll need to supplement your diet with calcium in other ways (such as dark, leafy greens). Plant-based diets are also linked to reduced risks of kidney disease and chronic kidney-related complications. When you don't eat meat, your kidneys have to do far less work to process protein and other nutrients, meaning they can stay healthier longer.

Your 50s and later is a time when you are more likely to experience weight gain – and when women, who are going through menopause, may have an increased risk of heart disease. Going vegan may help prevent this weight gain and the risk of heart disease. It can also help prevent and manage type 2 diabetes, which is most common in older adults.

The biggest health risk of going vegan has to do with muscle loss as a result of inadequate protein intake. Another disadvantage of a vegan diet is it is relatively low in energy-promoting mitochondrial nutrients such as B12, carnitine, coq10, and zinc, to name a few. Dysfunction in your mitochondria contributes to many chronic diseases, and it has been implicated in at least one theory of ageing. The vegan diet is largely absent or low in key nutrients that quench inflammation: omega-3 fatty acids. Some mitochondrial powerhouse foods such as salmon and liver/organ meats are not vegan. If you consider being a vegan, it will likely also require careful supplementation with mitochondria-promoting nutrients and omega-3 fatty acids. Vegans are often deficient in the essential omega-3 fatty acids, particularly the DHA and EPA subtypes. These are most notably found in fish, but you can consume them in a vegan-only diet by consuming products like spirulina and chlorella. A well-balanced plant-based diet should include proteins like pulses, seeds, nuts, beans, and quinoa. All of these offer plenty of protein.

Muscle loss with ageing typically occurs in people who have a high-calorie intake from processed foods as well as from a sedentary lifestyle. By making healthy diet choices and keeping up with your exercise routine, you shouldn't notice any difference in your muscle loss from that of a person who consumes meat.

Vitamin B12 deficiency is another major concern. B12 only comes from animal-based foods and is essential for maintaining our nervous system, DNA, red blood cell formation, glucose metabolism, regulating new cell growth, and aiding in our cognition. You can combat this by consuming foods fortified with B12 (such as breakfast cereals, certain plant milk, and some soy products). You can take a plant-based B12 supplement, too.

Calcium is essential for blood, bone, heart, dental, and nerve health. The most obvious source of calcium is dairy, but you can also get all the calcium you need from things like green, leafy vegetables. Broccoli and cabbage are two of the best – spinach also has lots of calcium, calcium-set tofu, kale, and sesame seeds. Oranges and figs are high in calcium as well. More vegetables can supply calcium, including bok choy, broccoli, Chinese cabbage, collards, and kale.

For heart protection, it's best to choose high-fibre whole grains and legumes, which are digested slowly and have a low glycemic index — that is, they help keep blood sugar levels steady. Soluble fibre also helps reduce cholesterol levels. Refined carbohydrates and starches like potatoes, white rice, and white-flour products cause a rapid rise in blood sugar, which increases the risk of heart attack and diabetes (a risk factor for heart disease). Nuts Are Also Heart-Protective. They have a low glycemic index and contain many antioxidants, vegetable protein, fibre, minerals, and healthy fatty acids. Walnuts, in particular, are a rich source of omega-3 fatty acids, which have many health benefits.

Compared with meat eaters, vegetarians tend to consume less saturated fat and cholesterol and more vitamins C and E, dietary fibre, folic acid, potassium, magnesium, and phytochemicals (plant chemicals), such as carotenoids and flavonoids. As a result, they're likely to have lower total and LDL (bad) cholesterol, lower blood pressure, and lower body mass index (BMI), all of which are associated with longevity and a reduced risk for many chronic diseases. The plant-based diet promotes health and longevity better than any other diet or lifestyle choice known to the medical field. A vegan diet can be a healthy and nutritious choice for many people, as it emphasizes whole plant-based foods that are rich in nutrients and low in saturated fat and cholesterol. In summary, a Plant-Based Diet Can turn Off Cancer Genes; slows aging, improves inflammation, weight, and vascular health, reverse heart disease and reduce the risk of type 2 Diabetes.

Even if you don't want to become a complete vegetarian, you can steer your diet in that direction with a few simple substitutions, such as plant-based sources. You can get many of the health benefits of being vegetarian without going all the way. For example, a Mediterranean eating pattern — known to be associated with longer life and reduced risk of several chronic illnesses — features an emphasis on plant foods with the sparing use of meat.

13. HEALTH BENEFITS OF SOCIAL

INTERACTION

Social support is essential for maintaining good mental health. Stay connected with family and friends, even if it's just a phone call or video chat. Social support is essential for maintaining good mental health. It--

- ***Helps You Cope With Stress.*** People who spend time with family and friends find healthier ways to cope with stress. People use their family and friends as a stress buffer, talking about their problems instead of seeking negative coping mechanisms like drinking alcohol, smoking or doing drugs.

- ***May Lengthen Your Life.*** An article in the American Society of Aging noted that older adults with larger social networks have a good episodic memory, better cognitive functions and a lower allostatic load, which is the wear and tear on the body and brain from being stressed. Having a good relationship with marital partners, adult children, siblings, and friends contributes to these positive health effects.

- ***Improves Psychological Well-Being.*** The emotional support provided by social ties enhances your psychological well-being. One study found that people who view their friends and families as supportive reported a greater sense of meaning in life and felt like they had a stronger sense of purpose.

- ***Is Good For Your Cardiovascular Health.*** Stress can actually encourage inflammation in the arteries, which is a precursor to atherosclerosis, or clogged arteries. Having good friends and a strong social support network can relieve stress. One study published in the Annals of Behavioural Medicine found that people who discussed difficult times in their lives had a lower pulse and blood pressure when they had a friend by their side.

Now that you've started reading books and getting materials to embark on this journey, it is important to note that you mainly need determination, commitment, discipline, consistency to achieve the success of keep a youthful body and enjoying a healthy and long life.

REFERENCES

1. https://www.verywellfit.com/why-does-weight-change-day-to-day- playfitness.com.au

2. https://www.ncbi.nlm.nih.gov/pmc/articles/PMC4712935/

3. https://www.medicalnewstoday.com/articles/biological-age-is-increased-by-stress-and-restored-upon-recovery-emb#What-the-study-on-biological-age-and-stress-revealed https://salmonhealth.com/blog/how-to-stay-young/

4. Exercise Right - Blog [Research Blog]

5. MedlinePlus (.gov)

6. Healthline.Com

7. californiamobility.com Do Vegans Age Better? Experts Share Their Thoughts

8. livekindly.com The Reason a Plant-Based Diet Has So Many Anti-Aging

9. health.harvard.edu Becoming a vegetarian

10. Vagaro.com

11. helloclue.com

12. drzenovia.com

13. thriva.com

14. ncbi.nlm.nih.gov

15. bbaesthetic.com

ABOUT THE AUTHOR

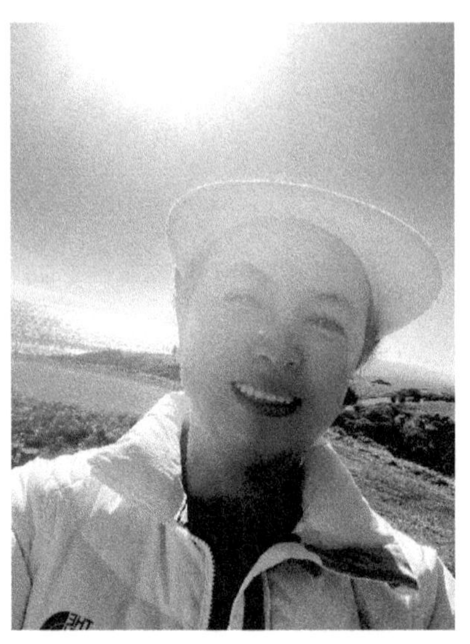

Susan Su holds a Ph.D. from U. C. Berkeley. She worked in the National Berkeley National Lab, consulted for National Aeronautics and Space Administration (NASA). She published many scientific papers at international and national journals. She is also a prolific author of fictions, non-fictions and screenplays.

SUSAN SU © 2023

www.ingramcontent.com/pod-product-compliance
Lightning Source LLC
Chambersburg PA
CBHW071519030726
47593CB00003B/1335